# KETO DIET RECIPES

## THE MOST MOUTH-WATERING POULTRY RECIPES TO GET LEAN AND STRONG

JOE CLAY

# Table of Contents

Introduction ................................................................................6
Poultry .......................................................................................11
   Duck Breast Salad ...............................................................12
   Turkey Pie ...........................................................................14
   Turkey Soup ........................................................................16
   Baked Turkey Delight .........................................................18
   Delicious Turkey Chili ........................................................20
   Turkey And Tomato Curry ..................................................22
   Turkey And Cranberry Salad ..............................................24
   Stuffed Chicken Breast .......................................................26
   Chicken And Mustard Sauce ...............................................29
   Delicious Salsa Chicken .....................................................31
   Delicious Italian Chicken ...................................................33
   Chicken Casserole ..............................................................35
   Chicken Stuffed Peppers ....................................................37
   Creamy Chicken ..................................................................39
   Different Chicken Casserole ...............................................41
   Creamy Chicken Soup .........................................................43
   Amazing Chicken Crepes ....................................................45
   Unbelievable Chicken Dish .................................................50
   Delicious Crusted Chicken .................................................52
   Cheesy Chicken ...................................................................54
   Orange Chicken ...................................................................56
   Chicken Pie .........................................................................58
   Bacon Wrapped Chicken .....................................................61
   So Delicious Chicken Wings ...............................................63
   Chicken In Creamy Sauce ...................................................65
   Delightful Chicken ..............................................................68
   Tasty Chicken And Sour Cream Sauce ................................70
   Tasty Chicken Stroganoff ...................................................72
   Tasty Chicken Gumbo .........................................................74
   Tender Chicken Thighs .......................................................76
   Tasty Crusted Chicken .......................................................78
   Pepperoni Chicken Bake .....................................................80

Fried Chicken ........................................................................ 82
Chicken Calzone .................................................................... 84
Mexican Chicken Soup .......................................................... 86
Spinach And Artichoke Chicken ............................................ 89
Chicken Meatloaf .................................................................. 91
Delicious Whole Chicken ...................................................... 94
Chicken And Green Onion Sauce .......................................... 96
Chicken Stuffed Mushrooms ................................................ 98
Chicken Stuffed Avocado ....................................................100
Delicious Balsamic Chicken .................................................102
Chicken Pasta .....................................................................104
Peanut Grilled Chicken ........................................................106
Conclusion ..............................................................................109

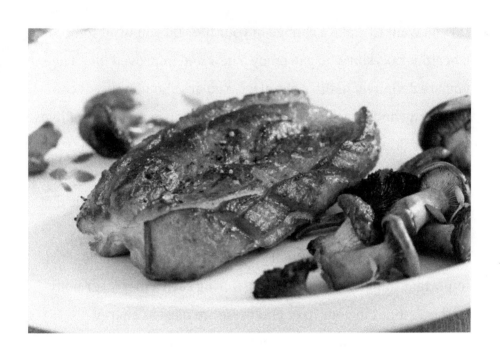

# Introduction

Do you want to make a change in your life? Do you want to become a healthier person who can enjoy a new and improved life? Then, you are definitely in the right place. You are about to discover a wonderful and very healthy diet that has changed millions of lives. We are talking about the Ketogenic diet, a lifestyle that will mesmerize you and that will make you a new person in no time. So, let's sit back, relax and find out more about the Ketogenic diet.

A keto diet is a low carb one. This is the first and one of the most important things you should now. During such a diet, your body makes ketones in your liver and these are used as energy.
Your body will produce less insulin and glucose and a state of ketosis is induced.
Ketosis is a natural process that appears when our food intake is lower than usual. The body will soon adapt to this state and therefore you will be able to lose weight in no time but you will also become healthier and your physical and mental performances will improve.
Your blood sugar levels will improve and you won't be predisposed to diabetes.

Also, epilepsy and heart diseases can be prevented if you are on a Ketogenic diet.

Your cholesterol will improve and you will feel amazing in no time. How does that sound?

A Ketogenic diet is simple and easy to follow as long as you follow some simple rules. You don't need to make huge changes but there are some things you should know.

So, here goes!

If you are on a Ketogenic diet you can't eat:

- Grains like corn, cereals, rice, etc
- Fruits like bananas
- Sugar
- Dry beans
- Honey
- Potatoes
- Yams

If you are on a Ketogenic diet you can eat:

- Greens like spinach, green beans, kale, bok choy, etc
- Meat like poultry, fish, pork, lamb, beef, etc
- Eggs
- Above ground veggies like cauliflower or broccoli, napa cabbage or regular cabbage
- Nuts and seeds
- Cheese
- Ghee or butter
- Avocados and all kind of berries
- Sweeteners like erythritol, splenda, stevia and others that contain only a few carbs
- Coconut oil
- Avocado oil
- Olive oil

The list of foods you are allowed to eat during a keto diet is permissive and rich as you can see for yourself.

So, we think it should be pretty easy for you to start such a diet.

If you've made this choice already, then, it's time you checked our amazing keto recipe collection.

You will discover 50 of the best Ketogenic Poultry recipes in the world and you will soon be able to make each and every one of these recipes.

Now let's start our magical culinary journey!
Ketogenic lifestyle...here we come!
Enjoy!

# Poultry

# Duck Breast Salad

*It's a tasty salad with a delicious vinaigrette!*

**Preparation time:** 10 minutes

**Cooking time:** 15 minutes

**Servings:** 4

**Ingredients:**

- 1 tablespoon swerve
- 1 shallot, chopped
- ¼ cup red vinegar
- ¼ cup olive oil
- ¼ cup water
- ¾ cup raspberries
- 1 tablespoon Dijon mustard
- Salt and black pepper to the taste

*For the salad:*

- 10 ounces baby spinach
- 2 medium duck breasts, boneless
- 4 ounces goat cheese, crumbled
- Salt and black pepper to the taste
- ½ pint raspberries
- ½ cup pecans halves

**Directions:**

1. In your blender, mix swerve with shallot, vinegar, water, oil, ¾ cup raspberries, mustard, salt and pepper and blend very well.
2. Strain this, put into a bowl and leave aside.
3. Score duck breast, season with salt and pepper and place skin side down into a pan heated up over medium high heat.
4. Cook for 8 minutes, flip and cook for 5 minutes more.
5. Divide spinach on plates, sprinkle goat cheese, pecan halves and ½ pint raspberries.
6. Slice duck breasts and add on top of raspberries.
7. Drizzle the raspberries vinaigrette on top and serve.

Enjoy!

**Nutrition:** calories 455, fat 40, fiber 4, carbs 6, protein 18

# Turkey Pie

*It's a great way to end your day!*

**Preparation time:** 10 minutes

**Cooking time:** 40 minutes

**Servings:** 6

**Ingredients:**

- 2 cups turkey stock
- 1 cup turkey meat, cooked and shredded
- Salt and black pepper to the taste
- 1 teaspoon thyme, chopped
- ½ cup kale, chopped
- ½ cup butternut squash, peeled and chopped
- ½ cup cheddar cheese, shredded
- ¼ teaspoon paprika
- ¼ teaspoon garlic powder
- ¼ teaspoon xanthan gum
- Cooking spray

*For the crust:*

- ¼ cup ghee
- ¼ teaspoon xanthan gum
- 2 cups almond flour
- A pinch of salt

- 1 egg
- ¼ cup cheddar cheese

**Directions:**

1. Heat up a pot with the stock over medium heat.
2. Add squash and turkey meat, stir and cook for 10 minutes.
3. Add garlic powder, kale, thyme, paprika, salt, pepper and ½ cup cheddar cheese and stir well.
4. In a bowl, mix ¼ teaspoon xanthan gum with ½ cup stock from the pot, stir well and add everything to the pot.
5. Take off heat and leave aside for now.
6. In a bowl, mix flour with ¼ teaspoon xanthan gum and a pinch of salt and stir.
7. Add ghee, egg and ¼ cup cheddar cheese and stir everything until you obtain your pie crust dough.
8. Shape a ball and keep in the fridge for now.
9. Spray a baking dish with cooking spray and spread pie filling on the bottom.
10. Transfer dough to a working surface, roll into a circle and top filling with this.
11. Press well and seal edges, introduce in the oven at 350 degrees F and bake for 35 minutes.
12. Leave the pie to cool down a bit and serve.

**Nutrition:** calories 320, fat 23, fiber 8, carbs 6, protein 16

# Turkey Soup

*It's a very comforting and rich soup!*

**Preparation time:** 10 minutes

**Cooking time:** 30 minutes

**Servings:** 4

**Ingredients:**

- 3 celery stalks, chopped
- 1 yellow onion, chopped
- 1 tablespoon ghee
- 6 cups turkey stock
- Salt and black pepper to the taste
- ¼ cup parsley, chopped
- 3 cups baked spaghetti squash, chopped
- 3 cups turkey, cooked and shredded

**Directions:**

1. Heat up a pot with the ghee over medium high heat, add celery and onion, stir and cook for 5 minutes.
2. Add parsley, stock, turkey meat, salt and pepper, stir and cook for 20 minutes.

3. Add spaghetti squash, stir and cook turkey soup for 10 minutes more.
4. Divide into bowls and serve.

Enjoy!

**Nutrition:** calories 150, fat 4, fiber 1, carbs 3, protein 10

# Baked Turkey Delight

*Try it soon! You will make it a second time as well!*

**Preparation time:** 10 minutes

**Cooking time:** 45 minutes

**Servings:** 8

**Ingredients:**

- 4 cups zucchinis, cut with a spiralizer
- 1 egg, whisked
- 3 cups cabbage, shredded
- 3 cups turkey meat, cooked and shredded
- ½ cup turkey stock
- ½ cup cream cheese
- 1 teaspoon poultry seasoning
- 2 cup cheddar cheese, grated
- ½ cup parmesan cheese, grated
- Salt and black pepper to the taste
- ¼ teaspoon garlic powder

**Directions:**

1. Heat up a pan with the stock over medium-low heat.

2. Add egg, cream, parmesan, cheddar cheese, salt, pepper, poultry seasoning and garlic powder, stir and bring to a gentle simmer.

3. Add turkey meat and cabbage, stir and take off heat.

4. Place zucchini noodles in a baking dish, add some salt and pepper, pour turkey mix and spread.

5. Cover with tin foil, introduce in the oven at 400 degrees F and bake for 35 minutes.

6. Leave aside to cool down a bit before serving.

Enjoy!

**Nutrition:** calories 240, fat 15, fiber 1, carbs 3, protein 25

# Delicious Turkey Chili

*This great keto dish is perfect for a cold and rainy day!*

**Preparation time:** 10 minutes

**Cooking time:** 20 minutes

**Servings:** 8

**Ingredients:**

- 4 cups turkey meat, cooked and shredded
- 2 cups squash, chopped
- 6 cups chicken stock
- Salt and black pepper to the taste
- 1 tablespoon canned chipotle peppers, chopped
- ½ teaspoon garlic powder
- ½ cup salsa verde
- 1 teaspoon coriander, ground
- 2 teaspoons cumin, ground
- ¼ cup sour cream
- 1 tablespoon cilantro, chopped

**Directions:**

1. Heat up a pan with the stock over medium heat.
2. Add squash, stir and cook for 10 minutes.

3.  Add turkey, chipotles, garlic powder, salsa verde, cumin, coriander, salt and pepper, stir and cook for 10 minutes.
4.  Add sour cream, stir, take off heat and divide into bowls.
5.  Top with some chopped cilantro and serve.

Enjoy!

**Nutrition:** calories 154, fat 5, fiber 3, carbs 2, protein 27

# Turkey And Tomato Curry

*You will make this in no time!*

**Preparation time:** 10 minutes

**Cooking time:** 20 minutes

**Servings:** 4

**Ingredients:**

- 18 ounces turkey meat, minced
- 3 ounces spinach
- 20 ounces canned tomatoes, chopped
- 2 tablespoons coconut oil
- 2 tablespoons coconut cream
- 2 garlic cloves, minced
- 2 yellow onions, sliced
- 1 tablespoon coriander, ground
- 2 tablespoons ginger, grated
- 1 tablespoons turmeric
- 1 tablespoon cumin, ground
- Salt and black pepper to the taste
- 2 tablespoons chili powder

**Directions:**

1. Heat up a pan with the coconut oil over medium heat, add onion, stir and cook for 5 minutes.

2. Add ginger and garlic, stir and cook for 1 minute.

3. Add tomatoes, salt, pepper, coriander, cumin, turmeric and chili powder and stir.

4. Add coconut cream, stir and cook for 10 minutes.

5. Blend using an immersion blender and mix with spinach and turkey meat.

6. Bring to a simmer, cook for 15 minutes more and serve.

Enjoy!

**Nutrition:** calories 240, fat 4, fiber 3, carbs 2, protein 12

# Turkey And Cranberry Salad

*It's healthy, it's fresh and very delicious! What are you still waiting for?*

**Preparation time:** 10 minutes

**Cooking time:** 0 minutes

**Servings:** 4

**Ingredients:**

- 4 cups romaine lettuce leaves, torn
- 2 cups turkey breast, cooked and cubed
- 1 orange, peeled and cut into small segments
- 1 red apple, cored and chopped
- 3 tablespoons walnuts, chopped
- 3 kiwis, peeled and sliced
- ¼ cup cranberries
- 1 cup cranberry sauce
- 1 cup orange juice

**Directions:**

1. In a salad bowl, mix lettuce with turkey, orange segments, apple pieces, cranberries and walnut and toss to coat.

2. In another bowl, mix cranberry sauce and orange juice and stir.
3. Drizzle this over turkey salad, toss to coat and serve with kiwis on top.

Enjoy!

**Nutrition:** calories 120, fat 2, fiber 1, carbs 3, protein 7

# Stuffed Chicken Breast

*This sounds really great, doesn't it?*

**Preparation time:** 10 minutes

**Cooking time:** 15 minutes

**Servings:** 3

**Ingredients:**

- 8 ounces spinach, cooked and chopped
- 3 chicken breasts
- Salt and black pepper to the taste
- 4 ounces cream cheese, soft
- 3 ounces feta cheese, crumbled
- 1 garlic clove, minced
- 1 tablespoon coconut oil

**Directions:**

1. In a bowl, mix feta cheese with cream cheese, spinach, salt, pepper and the garlic and stir well.
2. Place chicken breasts on a working surface, cut a pocket in each, stuff them with the spinach mix and season them with salt and pepper to the taste.

3. Heat up a pan with the oil over medium high heat, add stuffed chicken, cook for 5 minutes on each side and then introduce everything in the oven at 450 degrees F.
4. Bake for 10 minutes, divide between plates and serve. Enjoy!

**Nutrition:** calories 290, fat 12, fiber 2, carbs 4, protein 24

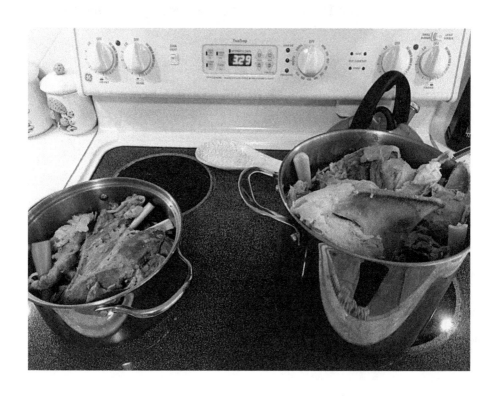

# Chicken And Mustard Sauce

*This is a magnificent combination of ingredients!*

**Preparation time:** 10 minutes

**Cooking time:** 30 minutes

**Servings:** 3

**Ingredients:**

- 8 bacon strips, chopped
- 1/3 cup Dijon mustard
- Salt and black pepper to the taste
- 1 cup yellow onion, chopped
- 1 tablespoon olive oil
- 1 and ½ cups chicken stock
- 3 chicken breasts, skinless and boneless
- ¼ teaspoon sweet paprika

**Directions:**

1. In a bowl, mix paprika with mustard, salt and pepper and stir well.
2. Spread this on chicken breasts and massage.
3. Heat up a pan over medium high heat, add bacon, stir, cook until it browns and transfer to a plate.

4. Heat up the same pan with the oil over medium high heat, add chicken breasts, cook for 2 minutes on each side and also transfer to a plate.

5. Heat up the pan once again over medium high heat, add stock, stir and bring to a simmer.

6. Add bacon and onions, salt and pepper and stir.

7. Return chicken to pan as well, stir gently and simmer over medium heat for 20 minutes, turning meat halfway.

8. Divide chicken on plates, drizzle the sauce over it and serve.

Enjoy!

**Nutrition:** calories 223, fat 8, fiber 1, carbs 3, protein 26

# Delicious Salsa Chicken

*Don't hesitate! Try this great keto dish today!*

**Preparation time:** 10 minutes

**Cooking time:** 1 hour and 15 minutes

**Servings:** 6

**Ingredients:**

- 6 chicken breasts, skinless and boneless
- 2 cups jarred salsa
- Salt and black pepper to the taste
- 1 cup cheddar cheese, shredded
- Vegetable cooking spray

**Directions:**

1. Spray a baking dish with cooking oil, place chicken breasts on it, season with salt and pepper and pour salsa all over.
2. Introduce in the oven at 425 degrees F and bake for 1 hour.
3. Spread cheese and bake for 15 minutes more.
4. Divide between plates and serve.

Enjoy!

**Nutrition:** calories 120, fat 2, fiber 2, carbs 6, protein 10

# Delicious Italian Chicken

*You should consider trying this Italian keto dish as soon as possible!*

**Preparation time:** 10 minutes

**Cooking time:** 1 hour

**Servings:** 6

**Ingredients:**

- 8 ounces mushrooms, chopped
- 1 pound Italian sausage, chopped
- 2 tablespoons avocado oil
- 6 cherry peppers, chopped
- 1 red bell pepper, chopped
- 1 red onion, sliced
- 2 tablespoons garlic, minced
- 2 cups cherry tomatoes, halved
- 4 chicken thighs
- Salt and black pepper to the taste
- ½ cup chicken stock
- 1 tablespoon balsamic vinegar
- 2 teaspoons oregano, dried
- Some chopped parsley for serving

**Directions:**

1. Heat up a pan with half of the oil over medium heat, add sausages, stir, brown for a few minutes and transfer to a plate.
2. Heat up the pan again with the rest of the oil over medium heat, add chicken thighs, season with salt and pepper, cook for 3 minutes on each side and transfer to a plate.
3. Heat up the pan again over medium heat, add cherry peppers, mushrooms, onion and bell pepper, stir and cook for 4 minutes.
4. Add garlic, stir and cook for 2 minutes.
5. Add stock, vinegar, salt, pepper, oregano and cherry tomatoes and stir.
6. Add chicken pieces and sausages ones, stir gently, transfer everything to the oven at 400 degrees and bake for 30 minutes.
7. Sprinkle parsley, divide between plates and serve.

Enjoy!

**Nutrition:** calories 340, fat 33, fiber 3, carbs 4, protein 20

# Chicken Casserole

*This could be your lunch today!*

**Preparation time:** 10 minutes

**Cooking time:** 40 minutes

**Servings:** 8

**Ingredients:**

- 1 and ½ pounds chicken breast, skinless and boneless and cubed
- Salt and black pepper to the taste
- 1 egg
- 1 cup almond flour
- ¼ cup parmesan, grated
- ½ teaspoon garlic powder
- 1 and ½ teaspoons parsley, dried
- ½ teaspoon basil, dried
- 4 tablespoons avocado oil
- 4 cups spaghetti squash, already cooked
- 6 ounces mozzarella, shredded
- 1 and ½ cups keto marinara sauce
- Fresh basil, chopped for serving

**Directions:**

1. In a bowl, mix almond flour with parm, salt, pepper, garlic powder and 1 teaspoon parsley and stir.
2. In another bowl, whisk the egg with a pinch of salt and pepper.
3. Dip chicken in egg and then in almond flour mix.
4. Heat up a pan with 3 tablespoons oil over medium high heat, add chicken, cook until they are golden on both sides and transfer to paper towels.
5. In a bowl, mix spaghetti squash with salt, pepper, dried basil, 1 tablespoon oil and the rest of the parsley and stir.
6. Spread this into a heatproof dish, add chicken pieces and then the marinara sauce.
7. Top with shredded mozzarella, introduce in the oven at 375 degrees F and bake for 30 minutes.
8. Sprinkle fresh basil at the end, leave casserole aside to cool down a bit, divide between plates and serve.

Enjoy!

**Nutrition:** calories 300, fat 6, fiber 3, carbs 5, protein 28

# Chicken Stuffed Peppers

*These will really impress your guests!*

**Preparation time:** 10 minutes

**Cooking time:** 40 minutes

**Servings:** 3

**Ingredients:**

- 2 cups cauliflower florets
- Salt and black pepper to the taste
- 1 small yellow onion, chopped
- 2 chicken breasts, skinless, boneless, cooked and shredded
- 2 tablespoons fajita seasoning
- 1 tablespoon ghee
- 6 bell peppers, tops cut off and seeds removed
- 2/3 cup water

**Directions:**

1. Put cauliflower florets in your food processor, add a pinch of salt and pepper, pulse well and transfer to a bowl.

2. Heat up a pan with the ghee over medium heat, add onions, stir and cook for 2 minutes.

3. Add cauliflower, stir and cook for 3 minutes more.

4. Add seasoning, salt, pepper, water and chicken, stir and cook for 2 minutes.

5. Place bell peppers on a lined baking sheet, stuff each with chicken mix, introduce in the oven at 350 degrees F and bake for 30 minutes.

6. Divide them between plates and serve.

Enjoy!

**Nutrition:** calories 200, fat 6, fiber 3, carbs 6, protein 14

# Creamy Chicken

*This is a really creamy and delicious keto chicken dish!*

**Preparation time:** 10 minutes

**Cooking time:** 1 hour

**Servings:** 4

**Ingredients:**

- 4 chicken breasts, skinless and boneless
- ½ cup mayo
- ½ cup sour cream
- Salt and black pepper to the taste
- ¾ cup parmesan, grated
- Cooking spray
- 8 mozzarella slices
- 1 teaspoon garlic powder

**Directions:**

1. Spray a baking dish, place chicken breasts in it and top each piece with 2 mozzarella slices.
2. In a bowl, mix parm with salt, pepper, mayo, garlic powder and sour cream and stir well.

3. Spread this over chicken, introduce dish in the oven at 375 degrees F and bake for 1 hour.
4. Divide between plates and serve.

Enjoy!


**Nutrition:** calories 240, fat 4, fiber 3, carbs 6, protein 20

# Different Chicken Casserole

*You must really make this tonight!*

**Preparation time:** 10 minutes

**Cooking time:** 45 minutes

**Servings:** 4


**Ingredients:**

- 3 cups cheddar cheese, grated
- 10 ounces broccoli florets
- 3 chicken breasts, skinless, boneless, cooked and cubed
- 1 cup mayo
- 1 tablespoon coconut oil, melted
- 1/3 cup chicken stock
- Salt and black pepper to the taste
- Juice of 1 lemon

**Directions:**

1.  Grease a baking dish with oil and arrange chicken pieces on the bottom.
2.  Spread broccoli florets and then half of the cheese.
3.  In a bowl, mix mayo with stock, salt, pepper and lemon juice.
4.  Pour this over chicken, sprinkle the rest of the cheese, cover dish with tin foil and bake in the oven at 350 degrees F for 30 minutes
5.  Remove foil and bake for 20 minutes more.
6.  Serve hot.

Enjoy!

**Nutrition:** calories 250, fat 5, fiber 4, carbs 6, protein 25

# Creamy Chicken Soup

*The taste is so amazing!*

**Preparation time:** 10 minutes

**Cooking time:** 20 minutes

**Servings:** 4

**Ingredients:**

- 3 tablespoons ghee
- 4 ounces cream cheese
- 2 cups chicken meat, cooked and shredded
- 1/3 cup red sauce
- 4 cups chicken stock
- Salt and black pepper to the taste
- ½ cup sour cream
- ¼ cup celery, chopped

**Directions:**

1. In your blender, mix stock with red sauce, cream cheese, ghee, salt, pepper and sour cream and pulse well.
2. Transfer this to a pot, heat up over medium heat and add celery and chicken.

3. Stir, simmer for a few minutes, divide into bowls and serve.

Enjoy!

**Nutrition:** calories 400, fat 23, fiber 5, carbs 5, protein 30

# Amazing Chicken Crepes

*These are even better than you can imagine!*

**Preparation time:** 10 minutes

**Cooking time:** 30 minutes

**Servings:** 8

**Ingredients:**

- 6 eggs
- 6 ounces cream cheese
- 1 teaspoon erythritol
- 1 and ½ tablespoons coconut flour
- 1/3 cup parmesan, grated
- A pinch of xanthan gum
- Cooking spray

*For the filling:*

- 8 ounces spinach
- 8 ounces mushrooms, sliced
- 8 ounces rotisserie chicken, shredded
- 8 ounces cheese blend
- 2 ounces cream cheese
- 1 garlic clove, minced

- 1 small yellow onion, chopped

*Liquids:*

- 2 tablespoons red wine vinegar
- 2 tablespoons ghee
- ½ cup heavy cream
- 1 teaspoon Worcestershire sauce
- ¼ cup chicken stock
- A pinch of nutmeg
- Chopped parsley
- Salt and black pepper to the taste

**Directions:**

1. In a bowl, mix 6 ounces cream cheese with eggs, parm, erythritol, xanthan and coconut flour and stir very well until you obtain a crepes batter.

2. Heat up a pan over medium heat, spray some cooking oil, pour some of the batters, spread well into the pan, cook for 2 minutes, flip and cook for 30 seconds more.

3. Repeat with the rest of the batter and place all crepes on a plate.

4. Heat up a pan with 2 tablespoon ghee over medium high heat, add onion, stir and cook for 2 minutes.

5. Add garlic, stir and cook for 1 minute more.

6. Add mushrooms, stir and cook for 2 minutes.

7. Add chicken, spinach, salt, pepper, stock, vinegar, nutmeg, Worcestershire sauce, heavy cream, 2 ounces cream cheese and 6-ounce cheese blend, stir everything and cook for 7 minutes more.

8. Fill each crepe with this mix, roll them and arrange them all in a baking dish.

9.  Top with 2 ounces cheese blend, introduce in preheated broiler for a couple of minutes.
10. Divide crepes on plates, top with chopped parsley and serve.

Enjoy!

**Nutrition:** calories 360, fat 32, fiber 2, carbs 7, protein 20

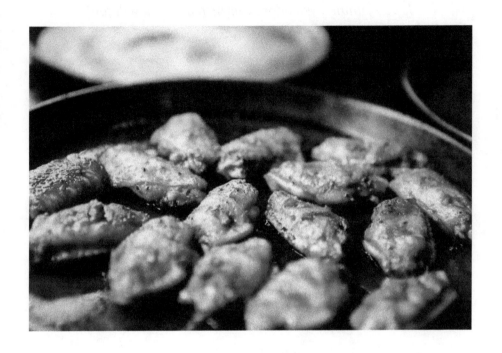

# Unbelievable Chicken Dish

*It's so yummy! We adore this dish and you will too!*

**Preparation time:** 10 minutes

**Cooking time:** 50 minutes

**Servings:** 4

**Ingredients:**

- 3 pounds chicken breasts
- 2 ounces muenster cheese, cubed
- 2 ounces cream cheese
- 4 ounces cheddar cheese, cubed
- 2 ounces provolone cheese, cubed
- 1 zucchini, shredded
- Salt and black pepper to the taste
- 1 teaspoon garlic, minced
- ½ cup bacon, cooked and crumbled

**Directions:**

1. Season zucchini with salt and pepper, leave aside few minutes, squeeze well and transfer to a bowl.

2. Add bacon, garlic, more salt and pepper, cream cheese, cheddar cheese, muenster cheese and provolone cheese and stir.

3. Cut slits into chicken breasts, season with salt and pepper and stuff with zucchini and cheese mix.

4. Place on a lined baking sheet, introduce in the oven at 400 degrees F and bake for 45 minutes.

5. Divide between plates and serve.

Enjoy!

**Nutrition:** calories 455, fat 20, fiber 0, carbs 2, protein 57

# Delicious Crusted Chicken

*You will soon end up recommending this amazing keto dish to everyone!*

**Preparation time:** 10 minutes

**Cooking time:** 35 minutes

**Servings:** 4

**Ingredients:**

- 4 bacon slices, cooked and crumbled
- 4 chicken breasts, skinless and boneless
- 1 tablespoon water
- ½ cup avocado oil
- 1 egg, whisked
- Salt and black pepper to the taste
- 1 cup asiago cheese, shredded
- ¼ teaspoon garlic powder
- 1 cup parmesan cheese, grated

**Directions:**

1. In a bowl, mix parmesan cheese with garlic, salt and pepper and stir.

2. Put whisked egg in another bowl and mix with the water.

3. Season chicken with salt and pepper and dip each piece into egg and then into cheese mix.

4. Heat up a pan with the oil over medium high heat, add chicken breasts, cook until they are golden on both sides and transfer to a baking pan.

5. Introduce in the oven at 350 degrees F and bake for 20 minutes.

6. Top chicken with bacon and asiago cheese, introduce in the oven, turn on broiler and broil for a couple of minutes.

7. Serve hot.

Enjoy!

**Nutrition:** calories 400, fat 22, fiber 1, carbs 1, protein 47

# Cheesy Chicken

*Your friends will ask for more!*

**Preparation time:** 10 minutes

**Cooking time:** 30 minutes

**Servings:** 4

**Ingredients:**

- 1 zucchini, chopped
- Salt and black pepper to the taste
- 1 teaspoon garlic powder
- 1 tablespoon avocado oil
- 2 chicken breasts, skinless and boneless and sliced
- 1 tomato, chopped
- ½ teaspoon oregano, dried
- ½ teaspoon basil, dried
- ½ cup mozzarella cheese, shredded

**Directions:**

1. Season chicken with salt, pepper and garlic powder.
2. Heat up a pan with the oil over medium heat, add chicken slices, brown on all sides and transfer them to a baking dish.

3. Heat up the pan again over medium heat, add zucchini, oregano, tomato, basil, salt and pepper, stir, cook for 2 minutes and pour over chicken.
4. Introduce in the oven at 325 degrees F and bake for 20 minutes.
5. Spread mozzarella over chicken, introduce in the oven again and bake for 5 minutes more.
6. Divide between plates and serve.

Enjoy!

**Nutrition:** calories 235, fat 4, fiber 1, carbs 2, protein 35

# Orange Chicken

*The combination is absolutely delicious!*

**Preparation time:** 10 minutes

**Cooking time:** 15 minutes

**Servings:** 4

**Ingredients:**

- 2 pounds chicken thighs, skinless, boneless and cut into pieces
- Salt and black pepper to the taste
- 3 tablespoons coconut oil
- ¼ cup coconut flour

*For the sauce:*

- 2 tablespoons fish sauce
- 1 and ½ teaspoons orange extract
- 1 tablespoon ginger, grated
- ¼ cup orange juice
- 2 teaspoons stevia
- 1 tablespoon orange zest
- ¼ teaspoon sesame seeds
- 2 tablespoons scallions, chopped

- ½ teaspoon coriander, ground
- 1 cup water
- ¼ teaspoon red pepper flakes
- 2 tablespoons gluten free soy sauce

**Directions:**

1. In a bowl, mix coconut flour and salt and pepper and stir.
2. Add chicken pieces and toss to coat well.
3. Heat up a pan with the oil over medium heat, add chicken, cook until they are golden on both sides and transfer to a bowl.
4. In your blender, mix orange juice with ginger, fish sauce, soy sauce, stevia, orange extract, water and coriander and blend well.
5. Pour this into a pan and heat up over medium heat.
6. Add chicken, stir and cook for 2 minutes.
7. Add sesame seeds, orange zest, scallions and pepper flakes, stir cook for 2 minutes and take off heat.
8. Divide between plates and serve.

Enjoy!

**Nutrition:** calories 423, fat 20, fiber 5, carbs 6, protein 45

# Chicken Pie

*This pie is so delicious!*

**Preparation time:** 10 minutes

**Cooking time:** 45 minutes

**Servings:** 4

**Ingredients:**

- ½ cup yellow onion, chopped
- 3 tablespoons ghee
- ½ cup carrots, chopped
- 3 garlic cloves, minced
- Salt and black pepper to the taste
- ¾ cup heavy cream
- ½ cup chicken stock
- 12 ounces chicken, cubed
- 2 tablespoons Dijon mustard
- ¾ cup cheddar cheese, shredded

*For the dough:*

- ¾ cup almond flour
- 3 tablespoons cream cheese
- 1 and ½ cup mozzarella cheese, shredded
- 1 egg

- 1 teaspoon onion powder
- 1 teaspoon garlic powder
- 1 teaspoon Italian seasoning
- Salt and black pepper to the taste

**Directions:**

1. Heat up a pan with the ghee over medium heat, add onion, carrots, garlic, salt and pepper, stir and cook for 5 minutes.
2. Add chicken, stir and cook for 3 minutes more.
3. Add heavy cream, stock, salt, pepper and mustard, stir and cook for 7 minutes more.
4. Add cheddar cheese, stir well, take off heat and keep warm.
5. Meanwhile, in a bowl, mix mozzarella with cream cheese, stir and heat up in your microwave for 1 minute.
6. Add garlic powder, Italian seasoning, salt, pepper, onion powder, flour and egg and stir well.

7.  Knead your dough very well, divide into 4 pieces and flatten each into a circle.
8.  Divide chicken mix into 4 ramekins, top each with a dough circle, introduce in the oven at 375 degrees F for 25 minutes.
9.  Serve your chicken pies warm.

Enjoy!

**Nutrition:** calories 600, fat 54, fiber 14, carbs 10, protein 45

# Bacon Wrapped Chicken

*The flavors will hypnotize you for sure!*

**Preparation time:** 10 minutes

**Cooking time:** 35 minutes

**Servings:** 4

**Ingredients:**

- 1 tablespoon chives, chopped
- 8 ounces cream cheese
- 2 pounds chicken breasts, skinless and boneless
- 12 bacon slices
- Salt and black pepper to the taste

**Directions:**

1. Heat up a pan over medium heat, add bacon, cook until it's half done, transfer to paper towels and drain grease.
2. In a bowl, mix cream cheese with salt, pepper and chives and stir.
3. Use a meat tenderizer to flatten chicken breasts well, divide cream cheese mix, roll them up and wrap each in a cooked bacon slice.

4. Arrange wrapped chicken breasts into a baking dish, introduce in the oven at 375 degrees F and bake for 30 minutes.
5. Divide between plates and serve.

Enjoy!

**Nutrition:** calories 700, fat 45, fiber 4, carbs 5, protein 45

# So Delicious Chicken Wings

*You will fall in love with this keto dish and you will make it over and over again!*

**Preparation time:** 10 minutes

**Cooking time:** 55 minutes

**Servings:** 4

**Ingredients:**

- 3 pounds chicken wings
- Salt and black pepper to the taste
- 3 tablespoons coconut aminos
- 2 teaspoons white vinegar
- 3 tablespoons rice vinegar
- 3 tablespoons stevia
- ¼ cup scallions, chopped
- ½ teaspoon xanthan gum
- 5 dried chilies, chopped

**Directions:**

1. Spread chicken wings on a lined baking sheet, season with salt and pepper, introduce in the oven at 375 degrees F and bake for 45 minutes.

2. Meanwhile, heat up a small pan over medium heat, add white vinegar, rice vinegar, coconut aminos, stevia, xanthan gum, scallions and chilies, stir well, bring to a boil, cook for 2 minutes and take off heat.
3. Dip chicken wings into this sauce, arrange them all on the baking sheet again and bake for 10 minutes more.
4. Serve them hot.

Enjoy!


**Nutrition:** calories 415, fat 23, fiber 3, carbs 2, protein 27

# Chicken In Creamy Sauce

*Trust us! This keto recipe is here to impress you!*

**Preparation time:** 10 minutes

**Cooking time:** 1 hour and 10 minutes

**Servings:** 4

**Ingredients:**

- 8 chicken thighs
- Salt and black pepper to the taste
- 1 yellow onion, chopped
- 1 tablespoon coconut oil
- 4 bacon strips, chopped
- 4 garlic cloves, minced
- 10 ounces cremini mushrooms, halved
- 2 cups white chardonnay wine
- 1 cup whipping cream
- A handful parsley, chopped

**Directions:**

1. Heat up a pan with the oil over medium heat, add bacon, stir, cook until it's crispy, take off heat and transfer to paper towels.
2. Heat up the pan with the bacon fat over medium heat, add chicken pieces, season them with salt and pepper, cook until they brown and also transfer to paper towels.
3. Heat up the pan again over medium heat, add onions, stir and cook for 6 minutes.
4. Add garlic, stir, cook for 1 minute and transfer next to bacon pieces.
5. Return pan to stove and heat up again over medium temperature.
6. Add mushrooms stir and cook them for 5 minutes.
7. Return chicken, bacon, garlic and onion to pan.
8. Add wine, stir, bring to a boil, reduce heat and simmer for 40 minutes.
9. Add parsley and cream, stir and cook for 10 minutes more.
10. Divide between plates and serve.

Enjoy!

**Nutrition:** calories 340, fat 10, fiber 7, carbs 4, protein 24

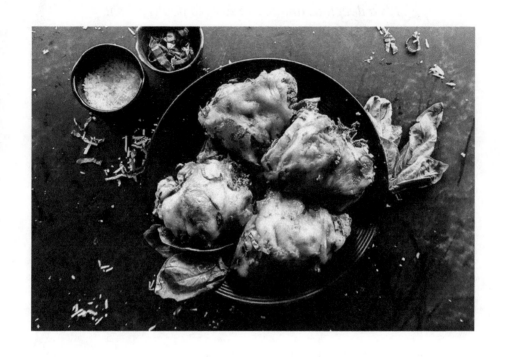

# Delightful Chicken

*It's a delicious and textured keto poultry dish!*

**Preparation time:** 10 minutes

**Cooking time:** 1 hour

**Servings:** 4

**Ingredients:**

- 6 chicken breasts, skinless and boneless
- Salt and black pepper to the taste
- ¼ cup jalapenos, chopped
- 5 bacon slices, chopped
- 8 ounces cream cheese
- ¼ cup yellow onion, chopped
- ½ cup mayonnaise
- ½ cup parmesan, grated
- 1 cup cheddar cheese, grated

*For the topping:*

- 2 ounces pork skins, crushed
- 4 tablespoons melted ghee
- ½ cup parmesan

**Directions:**

1.  Arrange chicken breasts in a baking dish, season with salt and pepper, introduce in the oven at 425 degrees F and bake for 40 minutes.
2.  Meanwhile, heat up a pan over medium heat, add bacon, stir, cook until it's crispy and transfer to a plate.
3.  Heat up the pan again over medium heat, add onions, stir and cook for 4 minutes.
4.  Take off heat, add bacon, jalapeno, cream cheese, mayo, cheddar cheese and ½ cup parm and stir well..
5.  Spread this over chicken.
6.  In a bowl, mix pork skin with ghee and ½ cup parm and stir.
7.  Spread this over chicken as well, introduce in the oven and bake for 15 minutes more.
8.  Serve hot.

Enjoy!

**Nutrition:** calories 340, fat 12, fiber 2, carbs 5, protein 20

# Tasty Chicken And Sour Cream Sauce

*You've got to learn how to make this tasty keto dish! It's so tasty!*

**Preparation time:** 10 minutes

**Cooking time:** 40 minutes

**Servings:** 4

**Ingredients:**

- 4 chicken thighs
- Salt and black pepper to the taste
- 1 teaspoon onion powder
- ¼ cup sour cream
- 2 tablespoons sweet paprika

**Directions:**

1. In a bowl, mix paprika with salt, pepper and onion powder and stir.
2. Season chicken pieces with this paprika mix, arrange them on a lined baking sheet and bake in the oven at 400 degrees F for 40 minutes.

3. Divide chicken on plates and leave aside for now.

4. Pour juices from the pan into a bowl and add sour cream.

5. Stir this sauce very well and drizzle over chicken.

Enjoy!

**Nutrition:** calories 384, fat 31, fiber 2, carbs 1, protein 33

# Tasty Chicken Stroganoff

*Have you heard about this keto recipe? It seems it's amazing!*

**Preparation time:** 10 minutes

**Cooking time:** 4 hours and 10 minutes

**Servings:** 4

**Ingredients:**

- 2 garlic cloves, minced
- 8 ounces mushrooms, roughly chopped
- ¼ teaspoon celery seeds, ground
- 1 cup chicken stock
- 1 cup coconut milk
- 1 yellow onion, chopped
- 1 pound chicken breasts, cut into medium pieces
- 1 and ½ teaspoons thyme, dried
- 2 tablespoons parsley, chopped
- Salt and black pepper to the teste
- 4 zucchinis, cut with a spiralizer

**Directions:**

1. Put chicken in your slow cooker.

2. Add salt, pepper, onion, garlic, mushrooms, coconut milk, celery seeds, stock, half of the parsley and thyme.

3. Stir, cover and cook on High for 4 hours.

4. Uncover pot, add more salt and pepper if needed and the rest of the parsley and stir.

5. Heat up a pan with water over medium heat, add some salt, bring to a boil, add zucchini pasta, cook for 1 minute and drain.

6. Divide on plates, add chicken mix on top and serve.

Enjoy!

**Nutrition:** calories 364, fat 22, fiber 2, carbs 4, protein 24

# Tasty Chicken Gumbo

*Oh. You are going to love this!*

**Preparation time:** 10 minutes

**Cooking time:** 7 hours

**Servings:** 5

**Ingredients:**

- 2 sausages, sliced
- 3 chicken breasts, cubed
- 2 tablespoons oregano, dried
- 2 bell peppers, chopped
- 1 small yellow onion, chopped
- 28 ounces canned tomatoes, chopped
- 3 tablespoons thyme, dried
- 2 tablespoons garlic powder
- 2 tablespoons mustard powder
- 1 teaspoon cayenne powder
- 1 tablespoons chili powder
- Salt and black pepper to the taste
- 6 tablespoons Creole seasoning

**Directions:**

1. In your slow cooker, mix sausages with chicken pieces, salt, pepper, bell peppers, oregano, onion, thyme, garlic powder, mustard powder, tomatoes, cayenne, chili and Creole seasoning.
2. Cover and cook on Low for 7 hours.
3. Uncover pot again, stir gumbo and divide into bowls.
4. Serve hot.

Enjoy!

**Nutrition:** calories 360, fat 23, fiber 2, carbs 6, protein 23

# Tender Chicken Thighs

*You'll see what we're talking about!*

**Preparation time:** 10 minutes

**Cooking time:** 45 minutes

**Servings:** 4

**Ingredients:**

- 3 tablespoons ghee
- 8 ounces mushrooms, sliced
- 2 tablespoons gruyere cheese, grated
- Salt and black pepper to the taste
- 2 garlic cloves, minced
- 6 chicken thighs, skin and bone-in

**Directions:**

1. Heat up a pan with 1 tablespoon ghee over medium heat, add chicken thighs, season with salt and pepper, cook for 3 minutes on each side and arrange them in a baking dish.
2. Heat up the pan again with the rest of the ghee over medium heat, add garlic, stir and cook for 1 minute.
3. Add mushrooms and stir well.

4. Add salt and pepper, stir and cook for 10 minutes.

5. Spoon these over chicken, sprinkle cheese, introduce in the oven at 350 degrees F and bake for 30 minutes.

6. Turn oven to broiler and broil everything for a couple more minutes.

7. Divide between plates and serve.

Enjoy!

**Nutrition:** calories 340, fat 31, fiber 3, carbs 5, protein 64

# Tasty Crusted Chicken

*This is just perfect!*

**Preparation time:** 10 minutes

**Cooking time:** 20 minutes

**Servings:** 4

**Ingredients:**

- 1 egg, whisked
- Salt and black pepper to the taste
- 3 tablespoons coconut oil
- 1 and ½ cups pecans, chopped
- 4 chicken breasts
- Salt and black pepper to the taste

**Directions:**

1. Put pecans in a bowl and the whisked egg in another.

2. Season chicken, dip in egg and then in pecans.

3. Heat up a pan with the oil over medium high heat, add chicken and cook until it's brown on both sides.

4. Transfer chicken pieces to a baking sheet, introduce in the oven and bake at 350 degrees F for 10 minutes.

5. Divide between plates and serve.

Enjoy!

**Nutrition:** calories 320, fat 12, fiber 4, carbs 1, protein 30

# Pepperoni Chicken Bake

*It's impossible not to appreciate this great keto dish!*

**Preparation time:** 10 minutes

**Cooking time:** 55 minutes

**Servings:** 6

**Ingredients:**

- 14 ounces low carb pizza sauce
- 1 tablespoon coconut oil
- 4 medium chicken breasts, skinless and boneless
- Salt and black pepper to the taste
- 1 teaspoon oregano, dried
- 6 ounces mozzarella, sliced
- 1 teaspoon garlic powder
- 2 ounces pepperoni, sliced

**Directions:**

1. Put pizza sauce in a small pot, bring to a boil over medium heat, simmer for 20 minutes and take off heat.
2. In a bowl, mix chicken with salt, pepper, garlic powder and oregano and stir.

3. Heat up a pan with the coconut oil over medium high heat, add chicken pieces, cook for 2 minutes on each side and transfer them to a baking dish.
4. Add mozzarella slices on top, spread sauce, top with pepperoni slices, introduce in the oven at 400 degrees F and bake for 30 minutes.
5. Divide between plates and serve.

Enjoy!

**Nutrition:** calories 320, fat 10, fiber 6, carbs 3, protein 27

# Fried Chicken

*It's a very simple dish you will like!*

**Preparation time:** 24 hours

**Cooking time:** 20 minutes

**Servings:** 4

**Ingredients:**

- 3 chicken breasts, cut into strips
- 4 ounces pork rinds, crushed
- 2 cups coconut oil
- 16 ounces jarred pickle juice
- 2 eggs, whisked

**Directions:**

1. In a bowl, mix chicken breast pieces with pickle juice, stir, cover and keep in the fridge for 24 hours.
2. Put eggs in a bowl and pork rinds in another one.
3. Dip chicken pieces in egg and then in rings and coat well.

4. Heat up a pan with the oil over medium high heat, add chicken pieces, fry them for 3 minutes on each side, transfer them to paper towels and drain grease.
5. Serve with a keto aioli sauce on the side.

Enjoy!

**Nutrition:** calories 260, fat 5, fiber 1, carbs 2, protein 20

# Chicken Calzone

*This special calzone is so delicious!*

**Preparation time:** 10 minutes

**Cooking time:** 1 hour

**Servings:** 12

**Ingredients:**

- 2 eggs
- 1 keto pizza crust
- ½ cup parmesan, grated
- 1 pound chicken breasts, skinless, boneless and each sliced in halves
- ½ cup keto marinara sauce
- 1 teaspoon Italian seasoning
- 1 teaspoon onion powder
- 1 teaspoon garlic powder
- Salt and black pepper to the taste
- ¼ cup flaxseed, ground
- 8 ounces provolone cheese

**Directions:**

1. In a bowl, mix Italian seasoning with onion powder, garlic powder, salt, pepper, flaxseed and parmesan and stir well.
2. In another bowl, mix eggs with a pinch of salt and pepper and whisk well.
3. Dip chicken pieces in eggs and then in seasoning mix, place all pieces on a lined baking sheet and bake in the oven at 350 degrees F for 30 minutes.
4. Put pizza crust dough on a lined baking sheet and spread half of the provolone cheese on half
5. Take chicken out of the oven, chop and spread over provolone cheese.
6. Add marinara sauce and then the rest of the cheese.
7. Cover all these with the other half of the dough and shape your calzone.
8. Seal its edges, introduce in the oven at 350 degrees F and bake for 20 minutes more.
9. Leave calzone to cool down before slicing and serving.

Enjoy!

**Nutrition:** calories 340, fat 8, fiber 2, carbs 6, protein 20

# Mexican Chicken Soup

*It's very simple to make a tasty keto chicken soup! Try this one!*

**Preparation time:** 10 minutes

**Cooking time:** 4 hours

**Servings:** 6

**Ingredients:**

- 1 and ½ pounds chicken tights, skinless, boneless and cubed
- 15 ounces chicken stock
- 15 ounces canned chunky salsa
- 8 ounces Monterey jack

**Directions:**

1. In your slow cooker, mix chicken with stock, salsa and cheese, stir, cover and cook on High for 4 hours.
2. Uncover pot, stir soup, divide into bowls and serve.

Enjoy!

**Nutrition:** calories 400, fat 22, fiber 3, carbs 6, protein 38

# Simple Chicken Stir Fry

*It's a keto friendly recipe you should really try soon!*

**Preparation time:** 10 minutes

**Cooking time:** 12 minutes

**Servings:** 2

**Ingredients:**

- 2 chicken thighs, skinless, boneless cut into thin strips
- 1 tablespoon sesame oil
- 1 teaspoon red pepper flakes
- 1 teaspoon onion powder
- 1 tablespoon ginger, grated
- ¼ cup tamari sauce
- ½ teaspoon garlic powder
- ½ cup water
- 1 tablespoon stevia
- ½ teaspoon xanthan gum
- ½ cup scallions, chopped
- 2 cups broccoli florets

**Directions:**

1. Heat up a pan with the oil over medium high heat, add chicken and ginger, stir and cook for 3 minutes.
2. Add water, tamari sauce, onion powder, garlic powder, stevia, pepper flakes and xanthan gum, stir and cook for 5 minutes.
3. Add broccoli and scallions, stir, cook for 2 minutes more and divide between plates.
4. Serve hot.

Enjoy!


**Nutrition:** calories 210, fat 10, fiber 3, carbs 5, protein 20

# Spinach And Artichoke Chicken

*The combination is really exceptional!*

**Preparation time:** 10 minutes

**Cooking time:** 50 minutes

**Servings:** 4

**Ingredients:**

- 4 ounces cream cheese
- 4 chicken breasts
- 10 ounces canned artichoke hearts, chopped
- 10 ounces spinach
- ½ cup parmesan, grated
- 1 tablespoon dried onion
- 1 tablespoon garlic, dried
- Salt and black pepper to the taste
- 4 ounces mozzarella, shredded

**Directions:**

1. Place chicken breasts on a lined baking sheet, season with salt and pepper, introduce in the oven at 400 degrees F and bake for 30 minutes.

2. In a bowl, mix artichokes with onion, cream cheese, parmesan, spinach, garlic, salt and pepper and stir.
3. Take chicken out of the oven, cut each piece in the middle, divide artichokes mix, sprinkle mozzarella, introduce in the oven at 400 degrees F and bake for 15 minutes more.
4. Serve hot.

Enjoy!


**Nutrition:** calories 450, fat 23, fiber 1, carbs 3, protein 39

# Chicken Meatloaf

*This is a special keto recipe we want to share with you!*

**Preparation time:** 10 minutes

**Cooking time:** 40 minutes

**Servings:** 8

**Ingredients:**

- 1 cup keto marinara sauce
- 2 pound chicken meat, ground
- 2 tablespoons parsley, chopped
- 4 garlic cloves, minced
- 2 teaspoons onion powder
- 2 teaspoons Italian seasoning
- Salt and black pepper to the taste

*For the filling:*

- ½ cup ricotta cheese
- 1 cup parmesan, grated
- 1 cup mozzarella, shredded
- 2 teaspoons chives, chopped
- 2 tablespoons parsley, chopped
- 1 garlic clove, minced

**Directions:**

1. In a bowl, mix chicken with half of the marinara sauce, salt, pepper, Italian seasoning, 4 garlic cloves, onion powder and 2 tablespoons parsley and stir well.
2. In another bowl, mix ricotta with half of the parmesan, half of the mozzarella, chives, 1 garlic clove, salt, pepper and 2 tablespoons parsley and stir well.
3. Put half of the chicken mix into a loaf pan and spread evenly.
4. Add cheese filling and also spread.
5. Top with the rest of the meat and spread again.
6. Introduce meatloaf in the oven at 400 degrees F and bake for 20 minutes.
7. Take meatloaf out of the oven, spread the rest of the marinara sauce, the rest of the parmesan and mozzarella and bake for 20 minutes more.
8. Leave meatloaf to cool down, slice, divide between plates and serve.

Enjoy!

**Nutrition:** calories 273, fat 14, fiber 1, carbs 4, protein 28

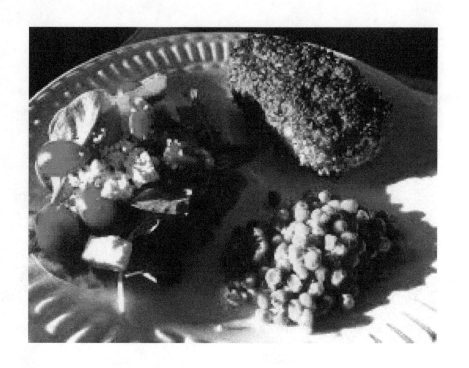

# Delicious Whole Chicken

*Cook this keto dish for a special occasion!*

**Preparation time:** 10 minutes

**Cooking time:** 40 minutes

**Servings:** 12

**Ingredients:**

- 1 whole chicken
- ½ teaspoon onion powder
- ½ teaspoon garlic powder
- Salt and black pepper to the taste
- 2 tablespoons coconut oil
- 1 teaspoon Italian seasoning
- 1 and ½ cups chicken stock
- 2 teaspoons guar guar

**Directions:**

1. Rub chicken with half of the oil, garlic powder, salt, pepper, Italian seasoning and onion powder.
2. Put the rest of the oil into an instant pot and add chicken to the pot.
3. Add stock, cover pot and cook on High for 40 minutes.

4. Transfer chicken to a platter and leave aside for now.

5. Set the instant pot on Sauté mode, add guar guar, stir and cook until it thickens.

6. Pour sauce over chicken and serve.

Enjoy!

**Nutrition:** calories 450, fat 30, fiber 1, carbs 1, protein 34

# Chicken And Green Onion Sauce

*Tell all your friends about this keto dish!*

**Preparation time:** 10 minutes

**Cooking time:** 27 minutes

**Servings:** 4

**Ingredients:**

- 2 tablespoons ghee
- 1 green onion, chopped
- 4 chicken breast halves, skinless and boneless
- Salt and black pepper to the taste
- 8 ounces sour cream

**Directions:**

1. Heat up a pan with the ghee over medium high heat, add chicken pieces, season with salt and pepper, cover, reduce heat and simmer for 10 minutes.
2. Uncover pan, turn chicken pieces and cook them covered for 10 minutes more.
3. Add green onions, stir and cook for 2 minutes more.

4.  Take off heat, add more salt and pepper if needed, add sour cream, stir well, cover pan and leave aside for 5 minutes.
5.  Stir again, divide between plates and serve.

Enjoy!

**Nutrition:** calories 200, fat 7, fiber 2, carbs 1, protein 8

# Chicken Stuffed Mushrooms

*It's a simple recipe you will like for sure!*

**Preparation time:** 10 minutes

**Cooking time:** 10 minutes

**Servings:** 6

**Ingredients:**

- 16 ounces button mushroom caps
- 4 ounces cream cheese
- ¼ cup carrot, chopped
- 1 teaspoon ranch seasoning mix
- 4 tablespoons hot sauce
- ¾ cup blue cheese, crumbled
- ¼ cup red onion, chopped
- ½ cup chicken meat, already cooked and chopped
- Salt and black pepper to the taste
- Cooking spray

**Directions:**

1. In a bowl, mix cream cheese with blue cheese, hot sauce, ranch seasoning, salt, pepper, chicken, carrot and red onion and stir.

2. Stuff each mushroom cap with this mix, place them all on a lined baking sheet, spray with cooking spray, introduce in the oven at 425 degrees F and bake for 10 minutes.
3. Divide between plates and serve them.

Enjoy!

**Nutrition:** calories 200, fat 4, fiber 1, carbs 2, protein 7

# Chicken Stuffed Avocado

*You will have to share this with all your friends!*

**Preparation time:** 10 minutes

**Cooking time:** 0 minutes

**Servings:** 2

**Ingredients:**

- 2 avocados, cut in halves and pitted
- ¼ cup mayonnaise
- 1 teaspoon thyme, dried
- 2 tablespoons cream cheese
- 1 and ½ cups chicken, cooked and shredded
- Salt and black pepper to the taste
- ¼ teaspoon cayenne pepper
- ½ teaspoon onion powder
- ½ teaspoon garlic powder
- 1 teaspoon paprika
- Salt and black pepper to the taste
- 2 tablespoons lemon juice

**Directions:**

1. Scoop the insides of your avocado halves and put the flesh in a bowl.
2. Leave avocado cups aside for now.
3. Add chicken to avocado flesh and stir.
4. Also add mayo, thyme, cream cheese, cayenne, onion, garlic, paprika, salt, pepper and lemon juice and stir well.
5. Stuff avocados with chicken mix and serve.

Enjoy!

**Nutrition:** calories 230, fat 40, fiber 11, carbs 5, protein 24

# Delicious Balsamic Chicken

*It's an easy dish you can make today!*

**Preparation time:** 10 minutes

**Cooking time:** 20 minutes

**Servings:** 4

**Ingredients:**

- 3 tablespoons coconut oil
- 2 pounds chicken breasts, skinless and boneless
- 3 garlic cloves, minced
- Salt and black pepper to the taste
- 1 cup chicken stock
- 3 tablespoons stevia
- ½ cup balsamic vinegar
- 1 tomato, thinly sliced
- 6 mozzarella slices
- Some chopped basil for serving

**Directions:**

- Heat up a pan with the oil over medium high heat, add chicken pieces, season with salt and pepper, cook until they brown on both sides and reduce heat.

102

- Add garlic, vinegar, stock and stevia, stir, increase heat again and cook for 10 minutes.
- Transfer chicken breasts to a lined baking sheet, arrange mozzarella slices on top, then top with basil.
- Broil in the oven over medium heat until cheese melts and then arrange tomato slices over chicken pieces.
- Divide between plates and serve.

Enjoy!

**Nutrition:** calories 240, fat 12, fiber 1, carbs 4, protein 27

# Chicken Pasta

*It's a very great dinner idea! This keto dish is superb!*

**Preparation time:** 10 minutes

**Cooking time:** 30 minutes

**Servings:** 4

**Ingredients:**

- 2 tablespoons ghee
- 1 teaspoon garlic, minced
- 1 pound chicken cutlets
- 1 teaspoon Cajun seasoning
- ¼ cup scallions, chopped
- ½ cup tomatoes, chopped
- ½ cup chicken stock
- ¼ cup whipping cream
- ½ cup cheddar cheese, grated
- 1 ounce cream cheese
- ¼ cup cilantro, chopped
- Salt and black pepper to the taste

*For the pasta:*

- 4 ounces cream cheese
- 8 eggs
- Salt and black pepper to the taste

- A pinch of garlic powder

**Directions:**

1. Heat up a pan with 1 tablespoon ghee over medium heat, add chicken cutlets, season with some of the Cajun seasonings, cook for 2 minutes on each side and transfer to a plate.
2. Heat up the pan with the rest of the ghee over medium heat, add garlic, stir and cook for 2 minutes.
3. Add tomatoes, stir and cook for 2 minutes more.
4. Add stock and the rest of the Cajun seasoning, stir and cook for 5 minutes.
5. Add whipping cream, cheddar cheese, 1 ounce cream cheese, salt, pepper, scallions and cilantro, stir well, cook for 2 minutes more and take off heat.
6. Meanwhile, in your blender, mix 4 ounces cream cheese with eggs, salt, pepper and garlic powder and pulse well.
7. Pour this into a lined baking sheet, leave aside for 5 minutes and then bake in the oven at 325 degrees F for 10 minutes.
8. Leave pasta sheet to cool down, transfer to a cutting board, roll and cut into medium slices.
9. Divide pasta on plates, top with chicken mix and serve.

Enjoy!

**Nutrition:** calories 345, fat 34, fiber 4, carbs 4, protein 39

# Peanut Grilled Chicken

*It's a Thai keto recipe worth trying!*

**Preparation time:** 10 minutes

**Cooking time:** 20 minutes

**Servings:** 8

**Ingredients:**

- 2 and ½ pounds chicken thighs and drumsticks
- 1 tablespoon coconut aminos
- 1 tablespoon apple cider vinegar
- A pinch of red pepper flakes
- Salt and black pepper to the taste
- ½ teaspoon ginger, ground
- 1/3 cup peanut butter
- 1 garlic clove, minced
- ½ cup warm water

**Directions:**

- In your blender mix peanut butter with water, aminos, salt, pepper, pepper flakes, ginger, garlic and vinegar and blend well.

- Pat dry chicken pieces, arrange them in a pan and pour the peanut butter marinade over it.
- Toss to coat and keep in the fridge for 1 hour.
- Place chicken pieces skin side down on your preheated grill over medium high heat, cook for 10 minutes, flip, brush with some of the marinades and cook them for 10 minutes more.
- Divide between plates and serve.

Enjoy!

**Nutrition:** calories 375, fat 12, fiber 1, carbs 3, protein 42

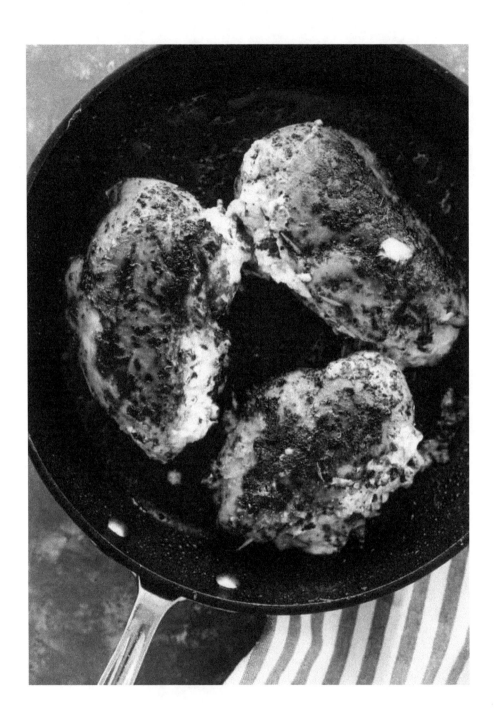

# Conclusion

This is really a life changing cookbook. It shows you everything you need to know about the Ketogenic diet and it helps you get started.

You now know some of the best and most popular Ketogenic recipes in the world.

We have something for everyone's taste!

So, don't hesitate too much and start your new life as a follower of the Ketogenic diet!

Get your hands on this special recipes collection and start cooking in this new, exciting and healthy way!

Have a lot of fun and enjoy your Ketogenic diet!

CPSIA information can be obtained
at www.ICGtesting.com
Printed in the USA
BVHW092149220221
600778BV00008B/917